"Thank you for the fantastic support you gave me to help my husband heal and get well. I appreciate your insight and spiritual strength."
Kim B.

"All these natural products and methods can sure be confusing, thanks for being someone I can talk to about it and get experience and knowledge from."
Tamara A.

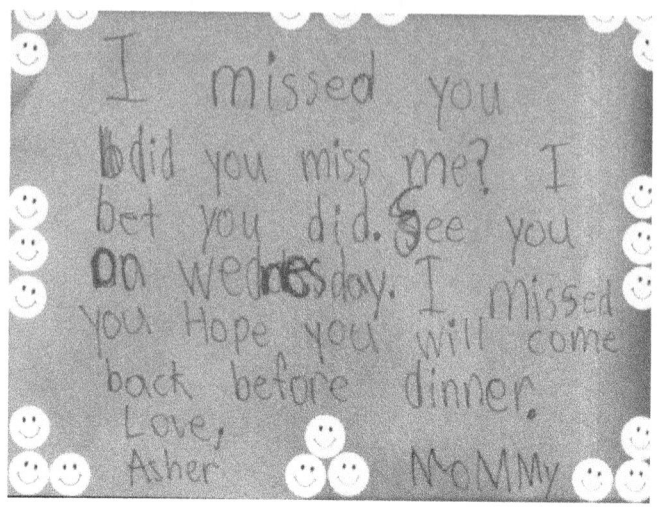

I missed you
b did you miss me? I
bet you did. See you
on wednesday. I missed
you Hope you will come
back before dinner.
Love,
Asher   MoMMy

I love you mommy. I have
ben praying formyou. I am
exided for you to feel
beter.

Support in Lyme

For

Families and Advocates

Janice Fairbairn

To my new circle of Lyme friends from California to Canada to Texas - Thank you for being like-minded and encouraging!

To the many incredible warrior mommies I know who have shown me how to be a mighty advocate.

To my earthly father, the best example of a warrior advocate I know, who doesn't give up. Thank you for your research and immense knowledge to recover my family.

I remain confident of this:
I will see the goodness of the LORD
in the land of the living.

Wait for the LORD;
be strong and take heart
and wait for the LORD.

(Psalm 27:13-14)

Table of Contents

Introduction

Depending on others isn't just hard for me, it's like kryptonite. The antitheses of the hardest things for me to do is to ask for help or to show my weakness. My parents did a great job of raising three girls to be independent and strong, almost to a fault.

This illness took not just my physical self and assurance of tomorrow (that was false to begin with), but it took my independence and strength. I have always been a pack mule, a rock, the strength in any storm. But who was my actual anchor? Was it my own strength or the Lord's? Is that why in the beginning of this trial I was hopelessly tossed about on the waves because the anchor in my own strength was not enough for the storm. I needed to remember my anchor in the Lord.

When I finally realized I had to let go of my independence and grasp the help that was being held out by my church community, family and friends, I was deeply rewarded. My mentor went from leader to best heart friend. She went from friendly sweet old lady to a grandma to my kids. God has grown beautiful new flowers of friendships and deepened roots on existing heart friends that helped me weather this storm.

Be honest with those around you, as honest as you possibly can. The rest you must be honest with the Lord as to not hold onto such toxic assets in your heart. Let go of the fear, the pain, the frustration, the confusion, the helplessness or it will fester and rot inside of you.

I hate the pain this is causing my kids and family. I despise that they have to watch me suffer, but you bring to mind the alternative and I am on my knees thanking you that it is me who gets to carry this burden. I am thankful that it is me who is suffering. For as long as it takes, let me carry this cross rather than for my husband or kids to suffer in it.

I wouldn't cast this upon even my worst enemy to hold and live. The suffering is too great to put upon even their bad deeds.

Thank you that I get to carry it. Thank you for sparing my family the anguish of having to live it, but only having to watch it.

Chapter 1 -To Spouse, Family Member, Friend

"As we pass through the land between, it is critical to recognize that not simply the hardship but also our reaction to the person we are in the hardship is forming us. With each discomfort we experience, our responses both reveal the person we are and set the trajectory for the person we are becoming. Whether we age with grace and poise or become bitter, resentful people is largely determined by our response to disappointment and the habits of response that often result." Jeff Manion The Land Between

One of the patients I met at the Lyme clinic was a little girl, 14 years old and her mom from California. She had been sick for years and had been to 42 doctors. 42 doctors!! I thought my 12 was bad, but 42? What causes traditional medicine to be such a bad listener? I've asked many Lymies I've met and the common denominator is that doctors aren't listening. People are not listening. Nobody believes them. Nobody understands.

I was shocked. Each of the doctors I saw also wanted to put me on antidepressants. There was no other medical explanation for why I wasn't eating or feeling so bad and losing weight. I must have been creating the whole illness in my head. And then I keep learning each patient experiences this with all of their doctors. For me this was the biggest surprise, I can come to terms with Lyme not being a well-known or popular illness, but to find out it is also unpopular and unknown in the medical world as well? That takes me and many other Lymies by storm.

Help your loved one navigate this and listen to them. Believe them. They need people around them that trust them and will help get doctors to listen, really listen.

Chapter 2 - Missing Out

I spent two semesters of college abroad, so upon my return, I was waiting tables in Chicago. Two young guys were trying to flirt and impress me. They were doing an impression of some characters that just made me look at them like they were crazy. They tried harder for a while using this technique to desperately get me to laugh or think them cool. It didn't work. Then a look passed between us that said "this girl is culturally clueless and these guys must be drunk on something."

You see, while I was gone from the country, I had missed the onset in our culture of two new characters that had hit like wildfire. I had missed the introduction of Beevis and Butthead. So, that day I thought those two guys were the crazy ones, they probably for the life of them couldn't figure out why I didn't know what they were doing and why it wasn't funny. Everybody knew Beevis and Butthead right? Wrong.

My husband and I began dating and attending his church and went through the welcome class there. The welcome class introduces you to the church and its doctrine, etc. Then I got a job and moved to NY for 9 months. Upon my return after 9/11, we got married and ended up staying in KS. That first Christmas, we were invited to a Christmas party of the newly married Sunday School class in the same church and one of the couples we had met in the welcome class came walking in with a baby. I had never seen them pregnant and they had a baby?

What does it mean to miss a year or two? How do you adjust to the holes that exist in your timelines when you check back in? How do you keep from feeling like you are missing out, not getting it?

I like being off the beat and path. My faith walk is so far out of bounds and that is fine with me, but culturally and relationally I am completely out of touch after losing 1 ½ years to Lyme. I don't want to be in the "know" culturally, but it still feels weird to not have a clue who was playing in or who won the Super Bowl two years in a row. I don't know who won Dancing with the Stars; I don't know the parent's names at school (let alone the kid's names). I came "back" and walked into church and everything looks different. We got a "revamp" look and new carpet and paint and a new logo and new coffee bar and it looks like a different place. I don't feel at "home" right away.

Missing out is a hard place to be. The illness is one thing, but to feel left out and missing out no one likes that. How can you keep your loved one plugged in spiritually and relationally and culturally? It's difficult, because some of that stuff seems so insignificant when your loved one is fighting for their life. On the other hand, it is great to get one's mind off such heavy things.

Even though it was difficult for me, plugging into a bible study group helped me connect with people and be in relationship. Help your Lymie to remain plugged in with friends, a support group, something. Keep them connected somehow with "things going on", a school newsletter, neighborhood newsletter, church bulletin, current prayer list, etc. These things can give a foothold into the year or season with a sense of what's going on, of not missing out.

Chapter 3 - Mean Janice

Gracia Burnam, a surviving missionary hostage who lost her husband right before the rescue, gave a talk at a women's retreat a few years ago on forgiveness. I'll never forget her talking about how the crisis in the jungle of the Philippines with her husband Martin initially gave both of them a different perspective. She said that "mean Gracia" came out in the woods with her captors, in complete contrast to Martin's grace and peace. I realized that through this crisis and valley, I too have been "mean Janice" at times especially to those I love because of my own frustration, exhaustion and lack of peace and fear.

There will be times, out of their control, that your loved one will just be cranky in the illness because of the pain, exhaustion and sheer terror of the length of the valley. At other times, it might be the lack of control, the need to be better faster, or a pity party. Try to help them discern it and give them a wide berth for the inner struggle of the soul. Character is being built in the valley. Pray for them. It's not you. It's the valley and the struggle of the heart. Kevin Malarkey discusses this in his book about his son's heavenly experiences "The Boy Who Came Back From Heaven."

My relationship with my wife Beth, was stretched to the breaking point. We are told to keep our eyes on Jesus , even in the midst of a raging storm. When we failed to do that, when we gave ourselves over to the flesh, the intensity of our lives made even the smallest issues loom larger than a mountain. I know that at times we were so caught up in our own pain, fears and physical exhaustion that we gave full vent to our baser selves. We have to be honest and admit that our relationship suffered great trauma, not only during Alex's first weeks in the hospital, but also for years after the accident.....We knew what the Bible said, but trying to live these words out in the center of the storm with nerves exposed and raw, we fell into sin – not sin that involved other people, we just weren't walking in love. We grew distant and irritable with each other.

It happens to all of us in the valley. The physical flesh is weakened and frail and tired and the enemy attacks further and we act out against one another. That is why having a support group is important. That is why having a counselor or pastor to meet with is integral in this process. Praying for one another, having someone to pray for you, having someone to pray for your loved one makes a difference. Support from others is an essential part of survival in the valley. You wouldn't go camping without the ability to make fire, cook food, find water, or find your way home. Don't go into this valley without the compass of prayer support and counseling.

Journal: Do not judge a girl on what you can see. She may be fighting cancer, or an incurable disease. She could be a girl in chronic pain. She comes in many forms. She is breathing, but she is hurting. She may look young, but she feels decades older. She smiles, but her heart sobs. She walks, she talks, she cooks, she cleans, she works when she can, and sometimes when she can't. She IS, but she IS NOT all at once. She is here, but a part of her is missing. She fights a battle you will never see. But if you can take a moment to look beyond that smile, you might see that the girl is me.
Caity B. - A Lyme Patient – 1-17-13

Chapter 4 - Judgment

In the book of Job, we see a good example of how judgment seems to come so easily to those looking out to the person in the valley. In chapter 8, one of Job's "friends" is speaking to him about how and why this must have happened to him. "When your children sinned against him, he gave them over to the penalty of their sin." He goes on to say to Job "Surely God does not reject a blameless man or strengthen the hands of evildoers."

In other words, all your children were killed because they were sinful and if you were blameless then God were surely not have done this to you. Ouch. Double ouch. Listen to Job's reply.

> *"But I have a mind as well as you; I am not inferior to you.....I have become a laughingstock to my friends, though I called on God and he answered – a mere laughingstock, though righteous and blameless! Those who are at ease have contempt for misfortune as the fate of those whose feet are slipping."*

Listen family and friends, it is "easy" to look at your loved one and try to dissect how this could have happened to them but it does no good. It's simple for other people in your family or your lives or church or community who are "at ease" and never fought this battle, to tell you what to do and how you got in the mess in the first place. People have no filter, no compassion until it happens to them. They have no clue. Don't take it to heart.

In the book Gathering Manna, the author mentions a story she heard once about a man who encountered a bull in the woods.

> *"The man would fight the bull till he could fight no more, then run to hide behind a rock. As long as the man stayed out of sight, the bull would leave him alone. However, after brief intervals, the man would rush from behind the rock to battle the bull again. Finally, an on-looker shouted, 'Hey, why don't you just stay behind the rock?' The wounded, harried man replied, 'There's a bear behind the rock!'"*

In this life we will have "trouble" Jesus proclaimed. It is a guarantee. Each of us will face trouble of a different kind and for some over and over again. But trouble is as certain as the sun rising in the east. This trouble is not predicated on sin, or the amount of sin, or previous sin or disobedience. It can be trouble for trouble's sake. This does not eradicate what the bible teaches us about consequences for sin. That still exists, but we don't get to judge what is a consequence and what is just plain ole trouble – only God knows that.

God will use valleys to build our character and refine us further to Him, but that does not mean as Job said, "though righteous and blameless." Job was not perfect, he was not without sin. But his intentions that God saw in his heart were to walk blamelessly.

Job knew "That which of these (bird/fish) does not know that the hand of the Lord has done this? In his hand is the life of every creature and the breath of all mankind.....To God belong wisdom and power; counsel and understanding are his. What he tears down cannot be rebuilt; those he imprisons cannot be released. If he holds back the waters, there is drought; if he lets them loose, they devastate the land."

Help your loved one have no guilt for this illness. No blame for this valley. It is what it is, just a heap of "trouble" that God can use to work out for good. He can build character; he can bring people to a saving knowledge of Him in the valley. NO blame, no judgment.

Journal Entry:
While on one hand, I have received more blessings than I could have ever asked for from the expected and unexpected places. I have also experienced extreme hurt and disappointment from

people judging our healthcare decisions, questioning our research and choices, needling us about money – all under the guise of caring about us.

This is not caring about us, that is standing in judgment against us. We may not be perfect people but the one thing people should know about us is that we don't move or walk forward without God's blessings. We do not act in willful disobedience against God in our lives. Every decision has been bathed in prayer and we have trusted God to open and shut doors he sees fit. Especially when we were tired and overwhelmed. Please Lord, help me in the future to do the same and not judge others and their decisions

I tell the kids often when they bicker "It's better to be loving than to be the one that is right." I need to take this to heart also for others. I cannot in turn judge why people have judged us or abandoned us in the crisis.

The thing about chronic Lyme is that most people are unaware of how serious it is and how sick one can become. Unless you saw me at my worst, you would not understand how closely I stood next to death's door. Also, I know some Lymies that "look" fine on the outside. Unless you look closely at the pain in their eyes you would not know how dysfunctional the physical body really is. For loved ones far away, it was very difficult to know how I was and how we were making the decisions we did.

Chapter 5 - Pray Without Ceasing

As Jesus crossed with his disciples into the Mount of Olives into the Garden of Gethsemane, he brought his closest, James, John and Peter with him farther into the garden and said to them "Pray that you will not fall into temptation." The second time he returned after praying he said to the three "Why are you sleeping? Get up and pray so that you will not fall into temptation."

If there is anything you can do without question for your loved one it is to pray. Pray for them, pray over them, pray with them, and organize prayer circles, prayer groups, and times of day to pray. Pray for them. Pray. Pray for wisdom and strength to do and say and support your loved one per God's will. Don't fall asleep on them. Don't lose your focus in your support of them.

When I quit drinking and got sober – there were many groups of friends that didn't walk through that with me because they and I were not comfortable with the faith component that was the trigger for the decision. Plus I was walking away from that lifestyle "completely", and that meant not hanging out with them anymore. But not knowing me after is like only reading the synopsis on the back cover of the book instead of reading the whole book.

Knowing my whole story is part of understanding what makes me what and who I am. Each chapter of the book is important. If those friends don't want to walk through this with you then they will be missing seeing the real you at the end – a chasm exists that now cannot be crossed.

There will be many, that maybe not for judgment's sake, but for the sake of fear and denial and sheer cowardess, will disappear for your loved one. Those who you thought you could count on and would help and be part of the rock that would hold you all up through this, they will falter. They will fail. Fear and denial are strong adversaries and for those who haven't fared a valley, the ability to walk away is easier. If they don't look it in the eye and see it, then they can't feel guilty for not helping, not being what they know they need to be. Doing the hard stuff for others takes grit and sacrifice. Some people just don't have the depth of soul to make it in the hard stuff. They just don't.

Journal: I am getting so frustrated. I am so tired of this. I'm tired of being sick. I'm tired of being in constant pain with NO relief ever. I'm tired of being exhausted 24/7 because I can't sleep more than two hours at night. I'm just tired of it ALL.

From the outside, my life looks normal. I'm working now; I am trying so hard to keep myself busy. When I'm busy, I don't have the time to think about how bad I feel. So while I am working, or hanging out with my friends, I try so hard not to focus on how miserable I am. But I always am miserable. I come home, and I cry myself to sleep because of pain. I come home and I feel so alone. I lost two very important people this year. My two best friends who said they would always be here. My life and my sickness got too much for them to handle, and like everyone else, they just disappeared. That hurts.

Caity B. - A Recovering Lymie– 18 yrs old

Your loved one will lose friends and feel betrayed. Look to the gifts in this. Those friends would have fallen off at some time, another hardship or for some other selfish reason to abandon. God is sifting them out for your loved one. He also works in the hearts of the saints to provide in surprising ways from people that you do not expect. Praise Him and thank Him for that and focus on the blessings.

God gives us many scriptures of encouragement in the role where you are – to watch a loved one suffer and suffer alongside them.

"For it has been granted to you on behalf of Christ not only to believe on him, but also to suffer for him." (Phil 1:20)

" For It is God who works in you to will and to act according to his good purpose." (Phil 2:13)

"Finally all of you, be like-minded, be sympathetic, love one another, be compassionate and humble. Do not repay evil with evil or insult with insult. On the contrary, repay with blessing, because to this you were called so that you man inherit a blessing." (1 Peter 3:8-11)

"Let us hold unswervingly to the hope we profess, for he who promised is faithful. And let us consider how we may spur one another on toward love and good deeds." (Hebrews 10:23-24)

Chapter 6 - DO

Take a look at this list to better understand our struggle before you begin to offer help:

- They are not crazy, they're not lazy, and it's not all in their head
- They are not stupid. They're under the influence (of the Lyme and toxins)
- They're on a special diet – honor it
- They are not ignoring you. They're reeling.
- Accept their decisions to leave the job or school or both
- Stop saying "well, you look healthy to me."
- They have been enduring this for months and years
- Treatment makes this hard and expensive.
- They don't have all the answers
- They are not bipolar

What things can you really do to help? This list is by no means complete, but it is a guideline of things and ideas. I wouldn't have even known some of these things that blessed me, but God laid them upon other's hearts and they were amazing. One particular lady in our church has been gathering a wholesome, uplifting movie collection over the years. She loans it out to people shut in and locked down after surgeries, illness, trauma, etc. What an interesting blessing and it was amazing to borrow.

You might also be the kind of spouse or family member who can do this all for your loved one. Don't. Let others help, it is part of the body of Christ and it blesses those who bless. Accept offers for help. Allow people to be in service for your whole family.

- Meals
- Prayer
- Cleaning/laundry
- Texts or notes of support and encouragement or scripture
- Help with kids – rides, play dates, entertainment
- Grown up time for their spouse – remove the burden for a moment
- Books
- Movies
- Newsletters to keep them plugged in
- Help journaling or blogging this valley for them
- A support group
- Donations or a fundraiser
- Counselor or therapist
- Prayer night – laying hands on in prayer, a prayer intervention, anointing with oil

Chapter 7 - What is an Advocate?

Blessed is the servant who loves his brother as much when he is sick and useless as when he is well and can be of service to him. And blessed is he who loves his brother as well when he is afar off as when he is by his side, and who would say nothing behind his back he might not, in love, say before his face. - St. Francis of Assisi

One fine spring Sunday morning, I was getting the kids ready for church (they were one and three). My husband leads worship at church, so he was already gone and I was trying to manage the chaos of diapers, high chairs – poop and church clothes. I had one watching Mickey Mouse and the other strapped in the high chair happily munching. So I thought, I'll outsmart myself and load up all the stuff in the car. We lived in not the greatest neighborhood and didn't have a garage, so I always locked up the house when I did this. The day before however, my husband and I had switched keys for some reason and I still had his keys. After I came back from loading the car, I couldn't find the house key on the ring to get back in the locked house.

I tried all the keys, none worked. I ran, now slightly panicking to the front door to try a different key, but the storm door was locked from the inside. So I banged on the window and tried to get the three year old to unlock the storm door to which he initially thought was a game then started crying because I couldn't get in. Then the one year old started crying and I started crying. It was 7:30 am on a Sunday, the neighbors were all sleeping, my husband wouldn't answer his cellphone because he was practicing singing for service and I didn't have a cellphone in my pocket anyway to call from.

So, I have to break in. I'm a momma and now both kids are crying and all instincts are on high alert. I am going to bust in that house somehow someway. You know, don't get in the momma bear's way. We lived in an old house with 6 foot tall windows and I thought, oh, my husband will kill me if I break one of those big windows to get in. So, I opted for the smaller back bathroom window. By now my adrenaline is on fire, I just stood sideways and lobbed my elbow at the window pane with all the strength I could muster. Why? Because I watched too many cop shows. Uh, it bounced off. Duh. I had to pick up a brick and break it to climb in.

So later, with kids calmed down and ice on my elbow and broken glass all over the back hallway, all things are right with the world once again.

Why tell that story? Well, that is the kind of advocate you need to be for your Lymie. Not the kind that irresponsibly locks their kids in the house, but the kind of advocate that would move heaven and earth to get in, to get the information, to help pull them out of the pit. The kind that is not afraid of a little bruised or cracked elbow. The kind that doesn't even need that brick but wouldn't be afraid to use it either.

An advocate in Roman times was "one called to aid". Webster's uses three different definitions I like

- To speak or write in favor of; support or urge by argument; recommend publicly
- A person who speaks or writes in support or defense of a person, cause, etc.
- A person who pleads for or in behalf of another; intercessor.

But let's go farther and see how the bible displays the use of advocate. We see in the Greek, it is used for one who pleads another's cause, who helps another by defending and/or comforting him.

Jesus uses it three times to refer to the Holy Spirit, John 14:16; 15:26; 16:7

"And I will ask the Father, and he will give you another Counselor to be with you forever"
"When the Counselor comes, when I will send to you from the Father, the Spirit of truth who goes out from the Father, he will testify about me."
"But I tell you the truth; it is for your good that I am going away. Unless I go away, the counselor

33

will not come to you, but if I go, I will send him to you."

It is applied to Christ in 1 John 2:1 "My dear children, I write this to you so that you will not sin. But if anybody does sin, we have one who speaks to the Father in our defense – Jesus Christ, the Righteous One."

Truly an advocate steps in when they see a need, defends and comforts the person publically, and pleads their case for favor and defense. That could be other family members or friends, with the doctors, with the insurance company, anybody standing in the way of peace for that person. Jesus is our advocate in heaven and he sent the Holy Spirit to be that advocate indwelt in our hearts. But on earth, in the Lyme battle, an earthly intercessor is priceless and important.

Romans 8:26 promises that "The Spirit helps us in our weakness, We do not know what we ought to pray for , but the spirit himself intercedes for us with groans that words cannot express." It also says in Eph 6:18 "and pray in the Spirit on all occasions with all kinds of prayers and requests."

Chapter 8 - How to be an Advocate

If you have been called to duty as an advocate for a loved one in this battle, remember that you have the Trinity in your corner. When you lack wisdom, ask God the Father.

"For the Lord gives wisdom; from his mouth come knowledge and understanding." (Proverbs 2:6)

When you question the road you are walking – Jesus Christ will come to your defense in heaven and advocate on your behalf.

Out of words to speak or pray – The Holy Spirit will fill in "with groans that words cannot express."

"Not a Fan" book, author Kyle Idelman says "Fans eventually get burned out from trying to live the Christian life out of their own efforts. If you are depending on your own strength to follow Christ you will soon find yourself drained and defeated. Followers of Jesus understand that it's a journey they were never to make alone. Instead we keep in step with the Spirit and he supernaturally gives us the strength and the power we need."

When you are sick and listening to doctor after doctor it begins to sound a bit like Charlie Brown. Remember, in the cartoon, the adults don't have actual words or voices. They say "Whah whah whah, whah whah whah." This phraseology is used in response to everything each child says to the adult. Listening to doctors and medical jargon sounds exactly like I'm standing in front of Charlie Brown's teacher hearing the instructions "whah whah whah". How do you discern that, how do you remember and digest it all and think straight when you are sick?

Being the gift and blessing of an advocate for someone relieves the burden. Shares the load. Believe me when I say, your Lymie needs someone to keep track of all that and voice questions and concerns where they have only exhausted silence. When they have no one to believe them, believe them. When they have no one to research, do the research. Take notes. Encourage them to exercise, eat right and look forward. Question everything and everyone. Help them keep focused where it matters, on God. And pray, pray, pray without ceasing.

During my struggle with Lyme, my husband was trying to hold together his own business and our family. Both our parents came to help and we had many a friend who lifted so many loads in our battle. The one thing we did not have was an advocate. At least a "full time" advocate. I took my dad to doctor appointments; friends would go and listen also at times. We were not alone in it, just didn't have at our employ a real full time supporter. I am the researcher and the advocate for the kid's health so it is a natural fit for me. Unfortunately, I couldn't look at the computer screen and read books so there was no research, no ability to dig deeper into therapies, doctors, experiences, chat rooms, etc. We had to trust that our prayer warriors were rousing the heavenlies and God would be my advocate.

In his book "The Land Between", Jeff Manion says it like this: "The land between is the perfect climate for transformational growth. In fact, no other soil in the world has the potential for producing life altering faith." It will produce transformational growth in anyone touching the valley and in the valley if they are willing. Even the advocate."

When I was in Las Vegas preparing to undergo CCSVI surgery to unclog the blood in my brain, I thought, "How did I get here – I don't know really anything about what I am about to do?" Later that afternoon, a fellow patient who had undergone the surgery called and put my mind at peace. The land between doesn't just produce life altering faith, it produces life altering trust. God comes through, his faithfulness is verified in the trial and it comes out proven.

In college I spent two semesters abroad and travelled quite a bit. My two travelling partners couldn't have been more polar opposite. One on the one hand had her "Let's go to Europe" book and had a set agenda. The second, however, could make friends with a lamppost and get invited to dinner and a private tour of a yacht. These opposing views made for interesting travel, neither was wrong. You have to have the guide book so you don't miss the high points, but going off book is also the way to meet the heart and soul of a culture.

Be the advocate who hits all the high places and does all the right things by the book, but also be the advocate who goes off book and gets knee deep in the swamp of this adventure letting God take you somewhere amazing also. There is no "by the book" in fighting Lyme. It attacks each one contrarily, heals differently for all who it inflicts. Being an advocate in this is going off road.

"Often God chooses to meet us with his blessing in a place we do not choose to be. He will bless us on the detour. He will bless us in the land between. Often the place of blessing is not our place of preference." "The Land Between".

In Romans 12:2-4 Paul reminds us to "Not conform to the pattern of this world, but be transformed by the renewing of your mind. Then you will be able to test and approve what God's will is – his good, pleasing and perfect will." He will guide you, he will be your captain advocate. Let him drive the ship.

There will be times of doubt, times of tremendous pressure and only an empty chasm of information and seemingly no map of where to go. "Beloved, whenever you are doubtful as to your course, submit your judgment absolutely to the Spirit of God, and ask Him to shut against you every door but the right one. Say, 'Blessed Spirit, I cast on thee the entire responsibility of closing against my steps any and every course which is not of God. Let me hear Thy voice behind me whenever I turn to the right hand or the left." From Paul, by Meyer from Streams in the Desert.

May the God of hope fill you with all joy and peace as you trust in him, so that you may overflow with hope by the power of the Holy Spirit. Romans 15:13

Chapter 9 - I'm a Parent and Have Lyme

Extraordinary afflictions are not always the punishment of extraordinary sins, but sometimes the trial of extraordinary graces. C.H. Spurgeon

Before the Lyme diagnosis my health was up and down, mostly down. I was tired all the time; I mean I couldn't keep my eyes open or get up to do anything during the day. I felt like a Mack truck had run me over countless times on top of the biggest hangover I had ever experienced times ten.

My daughter was four years old when I got sick. She was the one home with me all the time. We had her in afternoon preschool three days a week and by mid-term, we pulled her out because it was just too hard for my husband to drive her and I couldn't. So she was stuck with me. My son was six and in the first grade at school all day. It was just my daughter and I and the Lyme. She would play alone or watch movies and I would just lay there and sleep.

It would make her sad that I was so tired and couldn't play with her. She would periodically wake me to give me pictures she had drawn or notes she had written. She couldn't write much then, but the notes would usually say

"I want my mommy to not be sad or sick" or "I love mommy and I want her to feel better". It was heartbreaking.

Of all the regrets I have it is that I didn't "farm" her out more often when we were alone without grandparent help. I regret that she had to sit there alone at four years old and watch her mommy disintegrate right before her eyes. Still now at seven, she is still reeling from how sick I became. She is more clingy and needy to the extreme at times and cries uncontrollably also. Her ups and downs are more like an adolescent than a child.

My six year old son, since he was at school all day, would stick to me like glue on the weekends and didn't fall asleep well or go to school well in the mornings either. I would have to peel him off me to get him to go.

It's not like we didn't talk about it. We talked about it and prayed about it often. They were with us with when we went to church and the elders anointed me with oil and laid hands on me to pray for healing. In fact, after that event, my daughter, would cross the room and periodically lay her hands on me on the couch and pray for my healing. It's just too much for their little minds and emotions to process.

We prayed out their fears, gave my body over to the Lord, gave the illness over to God. I'm not sure what else I would have done differently except to have someone with our daughter more often in our house or outside it. But yet, because she was so clingy, I'm not sure that would have worked either.

What I do know, is that despite their fears and emotional mood swings since I was sick, their spiritual life and connection to God is thriving. What he did to their child size faith to grow it to such a dependence on Him was immense and transformational.

The boldness in which they pray and their understanding of scripture and prayer is amazing. I pray that each day we all are released of the shackles of fear more, the fear that it will return or take me. I know how I wrestle it and have to take those thoughts captive for Christ – how much more do they need that? On top of that, when a friend of ours died suddenly it transformed their thought process from "mommy is sick" to "mommy could die". We had to discuss often why we die and when and if I would.

> *"Let us not become weary in doing good, for at the proper time we will reap a harvest if we do not give up." (Galatians 6:9)*

No matter how bad I felt, no matter how bad a night it had been or how much sleep I had not had, The Lord awoke me morning after morning and gave me just enough strength to get out of bed, help the kids get ready for school, and eat breakfast with them. I tried to maintain the "routine" of our day which included making my son's lunch, reading the devotional and saying their blessing before school began. I look back even now and cannot imagine how I got that accomplished. It was only the Lord's strength and what he knew my kids needed.

Romans 5:3-4 "Not only so, but we also glory in our sufferings, because we know that suffering produces perseverance; perseverance, character; and character, hope. And hope does not disappoint us. "It is through this process described in the verse that each step and each day was sifted through. One day at a time. One thing at a time. In James 1:2-4 He says it like this "Consider it pure joy, my brothers and sisters, whenever you face trials of many kinds, because you know that the testing of your faith produces perseverance. Let perseverance finish its work so that you may be mature and complete, not lacking anything."

Chapter 10 - Being a Parent with Lyme

Ask for help with the cooking, laundry, housecleaning, grocery shopping – everything you can so you can hold tight to any time with your kids and give them some semblance of a routine or normal that they are used to. We still tried to have family game night, family movie night – anything we could for them.

I couldn't play and run and do all the things I used to in the yard with my very active son, but I would stand on the deck and throw the football to him in the yard over and over leaning on the railing at times just to be able to hold myself up. Again, this was not by my own strength, but God's alone.

Hold fast to him as the rock and anchor of your physical being as well as the spiritual one. I know just getting vertical and putting one foot in front of the other is a demanding task. The Lord will give you strength and sustain you beyond what you can accomplish.

"Therefore, he is able to save completely those who come to God through him" – Hebrews 7:25
"If you then, though you are evil, know how to give good gifts to your children, how much more will your Father in heaven give good gifts to those who ask him?" Matthew 7:11

"Every good and perfect gift is from above, coming down from the Father of the heavenly lights, who does not change like shifting shadows." James 1:17

"He who did not spare his own son, but gave him up for us all – how will he not also, along with him, graciously give us all things?" Romans 8:32

"What, then, shall we say in response to these things? If God is for us, who can be against us?" Romans 8:31

The Lord is able and willing to sustain and give you this gift of strength. But it does not come in waves with an overflow to put into my "account". This nourishment came moment by moment, minute by minute and day by day. I cannot believe it possible, but I pulled off two birthday parties with food and a clean house and entertaining during the worst of times. The brain fog has kept me from remembering how it even got accomplished. I also pulled off Christmas, Valentines, Easter and some of the school parties and field trips. I didn't, God did. Sometimes he gave me extra strength and sometimes it happened by my bible study group sending over a cleaning lady or someone showing up to do laundry, or someone to drive me to the field trip, but He did it. He accomplished it.

God knew exactly what I needed. He is able. He is willing. He is mighty to save.

In Psalm 27, David says in verse 5 "For in the day of trouble he will keep me safe in his dwelling; he will hide me in the shelter of his sacred tent and set me high upon a rock." As the Psalm goes on we reach my favorite verses and a promise I have clung to in this storm. Verse 13-14 say this:

> *"I remain confident of this; I will see the goodness of the Lord in the land of the living. Wait for the Lord; be strong and take heart and wait for the Lord."*

The New King James Version says it this way "I would have lost heart, unless I had believed". You cannot lose heart. You cannot beat yourself up for what you are not doing or what you cannot do or what your children are watching happen. You must believe and trust His goodness.

Follow this verse and cling to it as a parent.

First be confident of Him. Be confident in his strength, his faithfulness, his purpose and plan.

Second, look for the goodness in your life. Make a thankful list for yourself and your kids so they can see God answering prayers and providing in abundance. Psalm 31:19 says "how abundant are the good things that you have stored up for those who fear you" He stores them up. There is stored up goodness just for you. Help your kids see this fact and how good the Lord has been in your lives and this valley.

Make a Chronicle of Wonder. We make scrap books and take pictures and pay for soccer videos, but not a journal of answers to prayer. Memorialize what God is doing for your family and in each of your kid's lives, especially through this valley.

The third is the hardest for me. **Wait for Him.** Without the first two, the confidence and seeing the goodness, waiting is excruciating. There seems to be no purpose in waiting with the fruit of goodness and faithfulness.

Be Strong. It says in Psalm 28:7 "The Lord is my strength and my shield; my heart trusts in him and he helps me. My heart leaps for joy, and with my song I praise him." Oh, it pains me to even write it because overcoming the physical ailments of being a Lymie is HARD, hard, hard. Lean on his strength and go moment by moment.

Take Heart. The Message version says "let your heart take courage". David says in Psalm 31:14 "but I trust in you Lord, I say you are my God. My times are in your hands, deliver me" Your heart must have courage in the Lord to muster the physical strength. Your kids will know when your heart has lost the courage to go on, to fight for it. David says in Psalm 143 "Lord hear my prayer, listen to my cry for mercy; in your faithfulness and righteousness come to my relief....so my spirit grows faint within me; my heart within me is dismayed. I remember the days of long ago and I meditate on all your works and consider what your hands have done."

Finally, he says again to "Wait for the Lord" Why twice? Because he is asking us to examine our plans versus his plans, our purpose versus His. Rest in the confidence of knowing He is acting when you physically cannot. In Isaiah 46:10-11 "I make known the end from the beginning, from ancient times, what is still to come. I say 'my purpose will stand and I will do all that I please' From the east I summon a bird of prey; from a far-off land, a man to fulfill my purpose. What I have said, that I will bring about; what I have planned, that I will do."

How is any of this possible? Because God is not just with us, he is in us. The Holy Spirit who dwells in you is the strength and miracle that allowed Peter to walk on water. The Holy Spirit who raised Lazarus and Jesus from the dead. The Holy Spirit who gave the disciples strength and courage upon his departure. That Holy Spirit lives in you and can take charge of your physical and mental faculties. He can. And he will upon your permission. He is able.

In Isaiah 59:21 the Lord says "My spirit, who is on you will not depart from you." He also promises in Philippians

4:19 through the words of Paul "And my God will meet all your needs according to the riches of his glory in Christ Jesus."

One day, in this struggle an old hymn came to mind. I had to Google the verses because I could only remember the chorus.

Because he lives, I can face tomorrow
Because he lives, all fear is gone
Because I know he holds the future
My life is worth the living just because he lives

The last verse says "And then one day I'll cross the river, I'll fight life's final war with pain".

Is this where you are? In life's war with pain. In Romans 8:37-38 Paul says "No in all these things we are more than conquerors through him who loved us. For I am convinced that neither death nor life, neither angels nor demons, neither the present nor the future, nor any powers, neither height nor depth, nor anything else in all creation will be able to separate us from the love of God that is in Christ Jesus our Lord.

You can face tomorrow because He lives. Because we can bask in God's love for us through Christ. Because the Holy Spirit is in you waiting for you to unleash his power over your life physically, spiritually and emotionally. He is able.

Chapter 11 - Parenting a Lyme Child

Have you ever lost your child? I have with each of my kids a "lost" story that would compete for the banner "incompetent mommy". Just as I begin to type it I feel the sheer panic rising up in my soul. The terror that befalls the moment of recognition and searching and screaming.

This is the sheer terror and utter despair that washes over me the day I realize my kids have Lyme also. While in treatment for a month or so, I had met already dozens of patients from all across the country of all ages. One particular mom had a son with Asperger's who also had Lyme. She began to tell me of the strong connection between Lyme and autism.

My mind began to process through our journey with the kids health and then the Lord hit me with it "both kids have Lyme, you have to bring them here for treatment."

Do you know that moment, that moment before a "diagnosis" is handed out? That moment when you know you need to know, but for this moment and the next you could live on just wondering without the knowledge? Oh, how I wanted to live in that moment of not knowing longer. But then I realized, the only place not knowing was going to take me was to more hardship and more strife.

I didn't want my kids growing up with this ticking time bomb inside of them ready to go off at a moment's notice like it did in me. I had to hire the bomb squad and go in after this thing proactively and get it turned off.

Yes, the doctor said. Both kids had every bad critter I had. Yes some were active. That only meant one thing. They had gotten them all from me. You try to do the mental math; I wonder how long I've actually had Lyme since I don't remember a bite or an event. I had thought back to how long I had symptoms. This just put the timeline back another 7 years at least.

But how could we afford this? How could I have the strength to guide them to healing and recovery when I was still but a shell myself? How could we not? How could we keep them wrapped in duct-taped health plan and diet that were just masking the underlining problem?

If Lyme has caused all the problems they have and are having then it has to go and it has to go now.

He promises me and you in 2 Peter 3:9 "He is not slow in keeping his promise, as some understand slowness. Instead he is patient with you, not wanting anyone to perish, but everyone to come to repentance."

I have been reading through the book of Isaiah and the Lord says "So is my word that goes out from my mouth; it will not return to me empty, but will accomplish what I desire and achieve the purpose for which I sent it." Isa 55:11 It is for this very reason that I claimed promises for my kids and pray scripture over them every day multiple times a day; for strength, for healing, for wisdom. He word will not return to him empty. On the days I felt powerless in this fight for my own life and the life of my kids, this verse comforted me. I felt the power it gives to know that these prayers are transcending time and space and reaching to heaven and back.

From verse 8-10 in the same chapter, "For my thoughts are not your thoughts neither are your ways my ways, declares the Lord. As the heavens are higher than the earth, so are my ways higher than your ways and my thoughts than your thoughts." I cannot understand the suffering of my kids, but for some reason with my Lyme explosion and all my suffering and symptoms, I finally understand why we have had the behavior problems we have had through the years with the kids.

If they ever felt even a little bit of what I have felt physically, it would cause me irrational behavior too. I have such more compassion for their heart issues and what struggles every day of their little lives have been fighting to get out of this thing before we even knew its name.

"Forget the former things; do not dwell on the past. See, I am doing a new thing! Now it springs up; do you not perceive it? I am making a way in the wilderness and streams in the wasteland." Isaiah 43:18-19 He is doing a new thing. He is the only one who can make a way in the wilderness of parenting a child suffering through Lyme.

Chapter 12 - Slow Down

I can tell you what illness also does. It makes you slow down. It takes the hurry out of life as quick as you can blow the dandelions seeds off the stem. I spent my life prior to this planning the next thing without even finishing the thing in front of me. In "1000 Gifts", Ann Voskamp quotes a story of a pastor speaking at a funeral "I cannot think of a single advantage I've ever gained from being in a hurry. But a thousand broken and missed things, tens of thousands lie in the wake of all the rushing."

Let parenting in Lyme or parenting a Lymie teaches you to stop and not hurry anymore. No regrets for time unspent or things left undone in the rushing. Take time to be with your child, your kids, your family. Jesus says in John 16:22 "Now is your time of grief, but I will see you again and you will rejoice and no one will take away your joy....Very truly I tell you, my Father will give you whatever you ask in my name. Until now you have not asked for anything in my name. Ask and you will receive, and your joy will be complete."

Ask and claim the promises of healing and respite over your family. Ask and pray for time well spent. Ask and pray for the rushing to be gone from the habits of your life.

Thank Him in advance for his mercy and goodness in giving you these good things.

Phil 4:19 "And my God will meet all your needs according to the riches of his glory in Christ Jesus." He will beloved, he will meet all the needs you have and that you give to him. "Surely God is my salvation; I will trust and not be afraid. The Lord, the Lord himself, is my strength and my defense he has become my salvation." Isaiah 12: 2. Trust Him; let him become your strength and salvation in this storm.

As I type this section, college friends of mine have just found out recently that their 9 year old daughter's inoperable brain cancer is growing and not responding the treatment. I cannot fathom the anguish they must feel, but Jesus does. I cannot imagine facing the end of this life with my child but Jesus can. As he came to Bethany after Lazurus , his friend, had died. This is our Jesus. "When Jesus saw her weeping, and the Jews who had come along with her also weeping, he was deeply moved in spirit and troubled. 'Where have you laid him?' he asked. 'Come and see, Lord,' they replied. Jesus wept. John 11:33-34 The words translated deeply moved and troubled come from anguish. He has felt loss and sadness and mourning.

One of my dear friends in bible study, who was widowed years ago and left with their 2 small boys, had only 4 months from diagnosis to death of her husband. She described to me that in the stage of extreme anguish and mourning one day she was crying and Jesus gave her the picture of himself, Jesus crying with her, mourning the loss of her husband.

Death and mourning were not part of the plan. They are part of the fallen world. Part of the sin nature. Part of why Jesus came to pay the debt and take the keys of Hades forever and give us the free gift of eternal life.

Do you not know? Have you not heard? The Lord is the everlasting God, the Creator of the ends of the earth. He will not grow tired or weary, and his understanding no one can fathom.

He gives strength to the weary and increases the power of the weak. Even youths grow tired and weary, and young men stumble and fall; but those who hope in the Lord will renew their strength. They will soar on wings like eagles; they will run and not grow weary, they will walk and not be faint. (Isaiah 40:28-31)

He will not grow tired or weary. Not tired of the tears, not tired of the prayers for healing, not tired of the sleepless nights and doctor's visits and bills to be paid.

But now, this is what the Lord says—he who created you, Jacob, he who formed you, Israel:

"Do not fear, for I have redeemed you; I have summoned you by name; you are mine.

When you pass through the waters, I will be with you; and when you pass through the rivers, they will not sweep over you. When you walk through the fire, you will not be burned;

the flames will not set you ablaze...Since you are precious and honored in my sight, and because I love you......do not be afraid, for I am with you."
(Isaiah 43:1-4, 5)

Conclusion and Postscript

Journal: By no accident these are the songs that come to mind today prompted by the Holy Spirit.

"My strength is in you Lord, my hope is in you Lord, in you it's in you"

"You are the strength when I am weak, you are the treasure that I see, you are my all in all"

"Strength for today and bright hope for tomorrow – great is thy faithfulness"

Do I detect a theme here? God knows my inner struggle with weakness, with asking for help, with being dependent on others, with a constant state of helplessness. He answers the cry of my heart that I am trying to suppress, trying to ignore. Instead of attempting to squelch or quiet my insecurity, my vulnerability, to this weakness, he as my Lord and Savior who cares, wants me to embrace it. I thank Him for getting to experience His strength. Oh what a marvel it is to be held up by his right hand, to sense his strength on a minute by minute level day after day.

Great is His faithfulness, the joy and intimacy in which I know Him pales in comparison to the pain from this valley. He has rescued me from myself. I was a workaholic with no time for family, no time to smell the roses but with starry eyed achievement. I did used to be there, act there, want that – it is the only thing I was intentional about, in fact I thrived there Mach 4 with my hair on fire.

But he has used parenting, marriage and now chronic Lyme disease to utterly derail my plans, gut out, and tear out the roots that were so firmly planted in my life and DNA. He changed my direction.

One of my friends and I were just discussing the other day another workaholic friend and she so gently said 'you were so headed there before God changed your direction." Amen sister.

My journey and my valley are not over. Our family's battles continue but we have a winning record. We are chipping away at what Lyme has done in our home.

I am driving, I am reading, and I am writing. Most importantly, I am living. I am living, my eyes focused forward and upward. Trying to see all things He brings each day in light of the character building God is doing in our family.

We are still eating GFCFSF, but all the other sensitivities for the kids are gone. We eat goat's cheese now which is a delicacy in our house and we treasure it. The kids sleep through the night much better, way over half the time. The behavior problems have been severely diminished. My daughter doesn't complain of tummy aches anymore or launch into prepubescent "tearcapades" either.

If fact, I can't remember the last time she complained about a tummy ache. Wow. We have come a long way and as I write this, it is a good reminder to be thankful and continue the fight.

I have gained 25 lbs. back but still have about 5 to go and can't seem to put it on no matter how much GF dessert I eat (what a problem huh?). But my pants are no longer duct taped up and I can fit into most of my clothes again. I've even graduated away from the "butt pillow" which I had to use for over a year because I was so thin that it hurt to sit at the kitchen table in our wood chairs without padding.

When we have "regressions" with my son, I claim and remember these things He has accomplished and hold fast to the journey to fight and finish it off.

When I look in the mirror now I see a ton of more gray hairs, but I see life. I see my soul reflecting back a life that was worth fighting for and worth keeping.

My goal for myself and my kids is to live life to the full knowing that each breath is a gift from God. For us to use our talents and experiences to help others find hope and healing. In small measure, I pray for continued strength and for cow's cheese to re-enter our house to be devoured in late night snacks.

My son's goal is to someday eat Papa John's pizza. Maybe someday we will. But until then, I just found out a new pizza place down the street is serving gluten free pizza...

I would encourage each of you to journal this process. Document somehow, via Facebook, blog or writing how you survived and thrived in the valley. Let it be a testimony to others of God's faithfulness and goodness. Use this period in your life to help make His name great. Help other's struggling with Lyme or other debilitating illnesses or physical ailments. Tell Him to let Him use you to help others and to be that testimony. I call it being a Lyme evangelist. This Lyme disease is the most undiagnosed illness in our country. Help others identify and get on the right path. Pray for them. Encourage them.

Dear Friends, I pray that you may enjoy good health and that all may go well with you, even as your soul is getting along well. (3 John 2) I pray that the Lord will heal all your diseases (Psalm 103:3) and be your strength every morning and be your salvation in your distress. (Isaiah 33:2) I pray that for you who fear His name, the Sun of Righteousness will rise with healing in his wings. And you will go free, leaping with joy like calves let out to pasture. (Malachi 4:2) I pray that your suffering now is nothing compared to the glory God will reveal to you later. (Romans 8:18)

Glossary

Ammonia - is a compound of nitrogen and hydrogen with the formula NH3 . ammonia is both caustic and hazardous. It is a by product of the die off of Lyme disease and its co-infections.

Ammonia Toxicity - has been shown to induce swelling of astrocytes in the brain

Asperger's - is an autism spectrum disorder (ASD) that is characterized by significant difficulties in social interaction and nonverbal communication, alongside restricted and repetitive patterns of behavior and interests. It differs from other autism spectrum disorders by its relative preservation of linguistic and cognitive development. Although not required for diagnosis, physical clumsiness and atypical (peculiar, odd) use of language are frequently reported.

Autism Spectrum Disorder (ASD)- Autism, Asperger syndrome, pervasive developmental disorder not otherwise specified (PDD-NOS), childhood disintegrative disorder, and Rett syndrome, although usually only the first three conditions are considered part of the autism spectrum. These disorders are typically characterized by social deficits, communication difficulties, stereotyped or repetitive behaviors and interests, and in some cases, cognitive delays.

Autonomic Nervous System - is the part of the peripheral nervous system that acts as a control system, functioning largely below the level of consciousness, and controls visceral functions.[1] The ANS affects heart rate,digestion, respiratory rate, salivation, perspiration, pupillary dilation, micturition (urination), and sexual arousal. Most autonomous functions are involuntary but a number of ANS actions can work alongside some degree of conscious control. Everyday examples include breathing, swallowing, and sexual arousal, and in some cases functions such as heart rate.

Chronic cerebrospinal venous insufficiency (CCSVI or CCVI) - a term developed by Italian researcher Paolo Zamboni in 2008 to describe compromised flow of blood in the veins draining the central nervous system

Chronic Lyme Disease – Having Lyme disease more than 4 weeks (as defined by the CDC) and suffering severe debilitating pain and illness for prolonged period of time.

Co-infections – Other pathogens that can be carried with the Lyme spirochete into the body simultaneously that can also cause damage and fatalities. Babesia, Bartonella, Ehrlichia, Colorado Tick Fever, Tick Relapsing Fever, Q Fever, Flavivirus, Rocky Mountain Spotted Fever, West Nile Virus, Tularemia, Micoplasma

Die Off – The affect of the body processing the toxic out put from bacteria, viruses, parasites, yeasts, etc in the body. It has been likened to a hangover, some more severe than others.

Herxheimer- is a reaction to endotoxins released by the death of harmful organisms within the body. In holistic medicine, it is sometimes referred to as a healing crisis, as it may coincide with recovery from an infectious disease, or a course of detoxification. It resembles bacterial sepsis. A byproduct of the spirochetes causes this reaction. Typically, the death of these bacteria and the associated release of neurotoxins occurs faster than the body can remove the substances. It usually manifests within a few hours of the first dose of any treatment to kill off the spirochete. It manifests as fever, chills, rigor, hypotension,headache, tachycardia, hyperventilation, vasodilation with flushing, myalgia (muscle pain), exacerbation of skin lesions and anxiety.

Lyme - an infectious disease carried by ticks caused by bacteria of genus Borrelia

Lymie – Any person suffering from Chronic Lyme Disease

Neurotoxin – The extrement product of the spirochete in its life cycle. Mass amounts are produced when the spirochete "die off". They are an extensive class of exogenous chemical neurological insults which can adversely affect function in both developing and mature nervous tissue.

Post Lyme Syndrome - Most medical experts believe that the lingering symptoms are the result of residual damage to tissues and the immune system that occurred during the infection. The body's "memory" of having chronic lyme disease

Sepsis - is a potentially deadly medical condition characterized by a whole-body inflammatory state caused by severe infection. It is caused by the immune system's response to a serious infection, most commonly bacteria, but also fungi, viruses, and parasites in theblood, urinary tract, lungs, skin, or other tissues.

Spirochete - bacteria, most of which have long, helically coiled (spiral-shaped) cells. The other most commonly known spirochete is syphilis

Resources

Lyme:

The One Minute Cure – Cavanaugh

The Yeast Connection – Crook

Detoxify or Die – Rogers

Beating Lyme Disease – Jernigan

Everyday Miracles by God's Design – Jernigan

Alkalize or Die - Theodore A. Baroody

Spiritual:

31 Days of Praise – Warren and Ruth Meyers

Streams in the Desert – Cowman

Jesus Calling – Sarah Young

Jesus Today – Sarah Young

Circle Maker – Mark Batterson

Drawing the Circle – Mark Batterson

Uplifting and Encouraging Reading:

Not a Fan – Kyle Idleman

I Am Second - Doug Bender, Sterrett, McCoy

Beautiful Outlaw – Eldridge

George Mueller – autobiography

Gathering Manna – Sue Fallin

Who is this Man? – John Ortberg

If You Want to Walk on Water You Have to Get Out of the Boat – John Ortberg

Fearless – Max Lucado

He Still Moves Stones – Max Lucado

The Boy Who Came Back From Heaven – Kevin and Alex Malarkey

Heaven is for Real – Todd Burpo

90 Minutes in Heaven – Don Piper

In a Pit with a Lion on a Snowy Day – Mark Batterson

Online:

Just Living Like This With Lyme on Facebook

justlivinglikethiswithlyme.com

jpfairbairn/just-living-like-this-with-lyme on Pintrest

Be a Lyme Evangelist - Zazzle.com

www.lymeresearchalliance.org

Hansa Center for Optimum Health

www.mercola.com

Young Living Essential Oils

www.bachflower.com

www.ccsvi.org

Lyme Search Engine - powered by Google

https://sites.google.com/site/lymediseasemapproject/home

Chart of Symptoms

Head, Face, Neck:
- Headaches/Migraines
- Facial paralysis (like Bell's palsy)
- Tingling of nose, cheek, or face
- Stiff neck
- Sore throat, swollen glands
- Heightened allergic sensitivities
- Twitching of facial/other muscles
- Jaw pain/stiffness (like TMJ)
- Change in smell, taste

Digestive/excretory System:
- Upset stomach (nausea, vomiting)
- Irritable bladder
- Unexplained weight loss or gain
- Loss of appetite, anorexia

Eye, Vision:
- Double or blurry vision, vision changes
- Wandering or lazy eye
- Conjunctivitis (pink eye)
- Oversensitivity to light
- Eye pain or swelling around eyes
- Floaters/spots in the line of sight
- Red eyes
- Vertigo

Ears/Hearing:
- Decreased hearing
- Ringing or buzzing in ears
- Sound sensitivity
- Pain in ears

Musculoskeletal System:
- Joint pain, swelling, or stiffness
- Shifting joint pains
- Muscle pain or cramps

- Poor muscle coordination, loss of reflexes
- Loss of muscle tone, muscle weakness
  Respiratory/Circulatory Systems:
- Difficulty breathing. Night sweats or unexplained chills
- Heart palpitations
- Diminished exercise tolerance
- Heart block, murmur
- Chest pain or rib soreness
  Psychiatric Symptoms:
- Mood swings, irritability, agitation
- Depression and anxiety
- Personality changes
- Malaise
- Aggressive behavior / impulsiveness
- Suicidal thoughts (rare cases of suicide)
- Overemotional reactions, crying easily Disturbed sleep: too much, too little, difficulty falling or staying asleep
- Suspiciousness, paranoia, hallucinations
- Feeling as though you are losing your mind
- Obsessive-compulsive behavior
- Bipolar disorder/manic behavior
- Schizophrenic-like state, including hallucinations
  Neurologic System:
- Numbness in body, tingling, pinpricks
- Burning/stabbing sensations in the body
- Burning in feet
- Weakness or paralysis of limbs
- Tremors or unexplained shaking
- Seizures, stroke
- Poor balance, dizziness, difficulty walking
- Increased motion sickness, wooziness
- Lightheadedness, fainting Encephalopathy (cognitive impairment from brain involvement)
- Encephalitis (inflammation of the brain)

- Meningitis (inflammation of the protective membrane around the brain)
- Encephalomyelitis (inflammation of the brain and spinal cord)
- Academic or vocational decline
- Difficulty with multitasking
- Difficulty with organization and planning
- Auditory processing problems
- Word finding problems
- Slowed speed of processing

Cognitive Symptoms:
- Dementia
- Forgetfulness, memory loss (short or long term)
- Poor school or work performance
- Attention deficit problems, distractibility
- Confusion, difficulty thinking
- Difficulty with concentration, reading, spelling
- Disorientation: getting or feeling lost

Skin Problems:
- Benign tumor-like nodules
- Erethyma Migrans (rash)
- Eczema
- Odd odors or higher perspiration than normal (ammonia)

General Well-being:
- Decreased interest in play (children)
- Extreme fatigue, tiredness, exhaustion
- Unexplained fevers (high or low grade)
- Flu-like symptoms (early in the illness)
- Symptoms seem to change, come and go
- Low body temperature
- Other Organ Problems:
- Dysfunction of the thyroid (under or over active thyroid glands)
- Liver inflammation
- Bladder & Kidney problems (including bed wetting)

Reproduction and Sexuality
Females:
- Unexplained menstrual pain, irregularity
- Reproduction problems, miscarriage, stillbirth, premature birth, neonatal
- Death, congenital Lyme disease
- Extreme PMS symptoms
Males:
- Testicular or pelvic pain
Autoimmune Disorders:
- Acute Coronary Syndrome
- Fibromyalgia
- Chronic Fatigue Syndrome
- Hashimoto's Hypothyroidism
- Graves' Disease/Hyperthyroidism
- Rheumatoid Arthritis
- Krohns Disease
- Irritable Bowel Syndrome
- Sjogren's Syndrome
- Parkinsons'
- Multiple Sclerosis
- Alzheimer's
- Dimentia
- Lupus
- Depression
- Autism
- ADHD
- Aspergers
- Dyslexia
- Psychological Disorders – Obsessive Compulsive, etc.
- Meniere's
- TMJ
- Celiac
- Addison's Disease
- Diabetes

- Cushing's Disease
- Polycystic Ovary Syndrome
- Restless Leg Syndrome
- Schizophrenia

About the Author

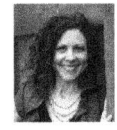 I am a 43 year old married, mother of 2. I discovered I had Lyme disease about 2012, after struggling most of 2011 with severe crashes and health crisis. I apparently had the slow workings of Lyme for over a decade because I gave everything I had to both my kids in the womb. They had been sick since birth and we had no idea what was going on with them. It has been a hard road, one that almost took my life as I hovered under 85 lbs, but it is one that has taught us all great life lessons and strengthened our faith.

As we were climbing out of our Lyme pit in 2013, I realized that God was compelling me to share my journey and give others who suffer a MEASURE OF HOPE.

In my previous life, I was a marketing and communications executive and then a work-from-home and stay-at-home mom. I have now become a PhD in health, healing, living right and all things Lyme. My passion is to see people embrace God's love and faithfulness by providing HOPE for their journey to healing. I love talking about health and healing to anyone who will listen. I adore my kids and how God has used our hardships to grow them into amazing young people with character and perseverance.

softcover book - http://www.amazon.com/author/janicefairbairn
Facebook - https://www.facebook.com/justlivinglikethiswithLYME
Blog - http://justlivinglikethiswithlyme.com/my-blog/
Twitter - https://twitter.com/lymeevangelist
Pintrest - http://www.pinterest.com/jpfairbairn/just-living-like-this-with-lyme/
YouTube - https://www.youtube.com/channel/UCul1VGlVLd6L0IjDwyPCOXg
Tumblr - http://janicelymeevangelist.tumblr.com/
ConnectPal - https://www.connectpal.com/janicefairbairn

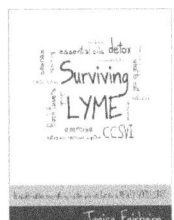

Surviving LYME

It might not be everything on the
planet, but it's a REALLY GOOD START.

Also sold separately or as an ebook.

- Compact and informative without being overwhelming
- Changing lifestyle choices in small chunks
- Must needs and haves for surviving LYME long term
- Do you want to win the battle or the WAR?

The top survival techniques we used at our house to live through the healing of LYME. Using natural biological methods as a framework, these helpful tips have become part of our family's healing and proactive stance against the Lyme monster.

How Many Different Ways to Heal? Let Me Count Thy Ways.......

Over the dozens of Lymies I've met through the past few years, there are common themed questions and areas that come up the most. I've done my best to document various methods of healing, helping, and surviving LYME disease.

A compilation of different methods used to heal, survive and treat Lyme disease based on our family's experience using non-traditional methods of biological medicine.

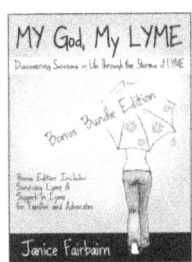

My God, My LYME

Discovering Success in Life
Through the Storms of LYME
- Bonus Bundle

Also sold separately or as an ebook.

Prepare for a Radical Battlefield. Includes Support in Lyme for Families and Advocates and Surviving Lyme.

Be inspired and encouraged by a true journey of faith through LYME. It's an amazing and real life success story. You can't help but be uplifted and gain strength from reading the story of one mom's compelling journey from the brink of death to healing and restoration for herself and her children from LYME.

Giving people the resources and HOPE they need for healing and how to live until they get there. Whether chronically ill with Lyme, already on your path to healing, or if you have conquered the mountain – this is for you.

- Discovering Success in Life out of the Storms of LYME.
- Be Inspired and Encouraged by this Journey of Faith
- Envision and Experience Whole Body Healing
- Prepare for a Radical Battlefield
- Get the Emotional and Spiritual Awakening You Desperately Need

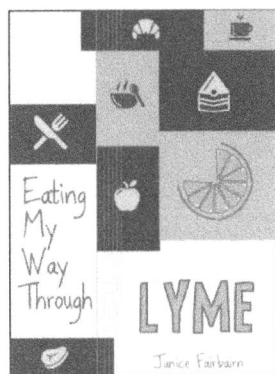

Don't Eat the Cardboard.

A Journey Eating My Way Through Lyme.

Available 2014 ebook.

www.selz.com

It is so hard to get well and get healthy at the same time.

I know going gluten free or dairy free just makes some of your head's spin. We've been gluten free, soy free and dairy free for almost 10 years now. These are adapted recipes and found recipes and combined recipes I've collected over the years to make our family happy and well fed. You don't have to do the research, you don't have to look for 5 years for a bread recipe that works or a pizza crust recipe your kids will eat – they are all in this collection. I am not a gormet cook, I'm just a mom who wanted to find recipes that worked without too much effort and that my family would enjoy. Your future in gluten free does not have to be bleak – you don't have to eat food that tastes like cardboard the rest of your life!!

https://justlivinglikethiswithlyme.selz.com/item/548b40d3b798720bbc12c742?mode =edit